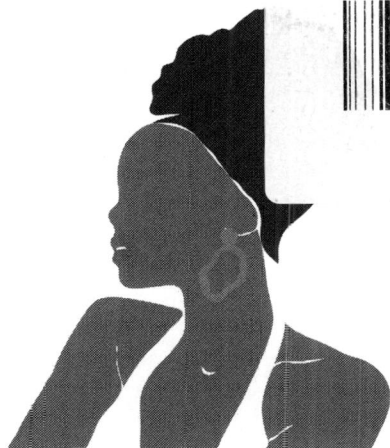

BlaCk
Hair Care
Journal

Get to know your hair, establish a successful hair care routine, and reach your hair goals.

This journal belongs to:

_____

_____

_____

_____

Healthy Hair Declaration:

_____

_____

_____

_____

_____

_____

_____

Order of Contents

About
How to Use
Definitions
Tips
Hair Profile
Daily Hair Tracker
Wash Days
Time to Switch it up!
Chemical Processes
Protective Styles
Cuts and Trims
Supplements
3 Month Check In
6 Month Check In
9 Month Check In
Final Check In
Ultimate Hair Care Regime

About

This simple, but extensive hair care journal will keep track of your hair care needs and journey you through a minimum of one years' worth of hair care. You will log your wash days, length checks, protective styles, supplements, chemical processes, cuts, and more, all while learning more about your hair along the way.

This book will help you to understand the methods of washing, conditioning, styling, and the products and tools that work for your particular hair. Regardless of what your hair goals are; be it longer, thicker, moisturized, curlier, shinier, or stronger hair, etc. this book will help you to recognize the things that you do (or don't do) in your hair care regime that are either pushing you closer to or further away from where you want to be.

All hair is equally beautiful,
but not all hair can be treated equally.

You can watch all of the tutorials in the world, however you still need to try them out to see if they will work for your hair! For hair to thrive, knowledge is required and hair knowledge is gained through experience in the form of trial and error.

Whether your hair is natural, dyed or chemically treated, with the guidance provided in this book, you will be well on your way to building a successful hair care routine and reaching your healthy hair goals!

How to Use

Please read through the definitions and tips provided.

Hair Profile: An overview of the current state of your hair. Carefully fill this in, making a note of your goals, problem areas and hair length - you will refer back to this later.

Daily Hair Tracker: You have creative license to log your shampoo days, wash days, supplements, moisturizing days, treatments, chemical processes. The legend can be letters, shapes or whatever you want. e.g. M = Moisturize and A = Ayurveda treatment.

Wash Day: Log 60 wash days, comprehensively specify the process, products, tools used, and also the results.

Chemical Processing: A place to comprehensively specify the process, products, tools used, and the results of your chemical treatment. You can log up to 8 processes.

Protective Styling: You can log up to 12 protective styles, how you prepped your hair and the condition of your hair after.

Cuts and Trims: You can log up to 12 cuts or trims.

Supplements: You can log the information of up to 11 supplements you have taken and the results/side effects.

Check Ins: Similar to the hair profile, a place to quickly update the quarterly condition and length of your hair, what has improved, and what still needs to be improved. Remember to set a reminder to fill it in!

Definitions

Density – The amount of hair growing out of the scalp. On average we have 80,000 to 120,000 hair strands. Lower density is not usually indicative of health however in some instances it can be, such as when we are nutritionally deficient or undergoing treatments such as chemotherapy. A way **test the density** is to put your hair in a pony tail. If the ponytail circumference is less than 2 inches, you have low density, if 2 to 3 inches, you have medium density, if any higher, then you have high density. The thickness of individual strands can affect this result.

Porosity – Your hair's ability to take in moisture. High porosity (porous) hair has more holes in the cuticle, this allows the hair to easily absorb moisture from water, conditioners and moisturizers. Low porosity hair has less holes, is tightly locked and struggles to absorb water. Even when wet, it can feel dry. You can **test porosity** by putting a strand of hair in water. If the hair floats, the hair has low porosity, if it sinks, high porosity. High porosity hair can get dry quickly however, moisture can be locked in with serums, oils and butters. Low porosity hair works well with heat treatments such as steaming, this enables the hair cuticle to open and draw in moisture. It needs clarifying shampoos as product easily builds up and makes the hair dull and dry. Chemical processing such as relaxers and dyes make hair porous. Protein treatments work well for high porosity hair but not so well for low porosity hair.

Thickness – The width of a single strand of hair. A person can have low hair density but high thickness. You can **test hair thickness** by comparing it to a piece of thread, if the strand is thinner, then you have fine hair, if it has the same thickness then you have thick hair, if thicker then your hair is coarse.

Type – Hair types show your curl pattern, there are four groups: 1 = Straight, 2 = Wavy, 3 - Curly, 4 = Coily. The letters a, b and c determine the texture; 'a' being looser, and 'c' being the tightest texture for that group. Some people profess to have type 5 hair.

TIPS

Ayurveda – There are many recipes using natural herbs and spices such as amla, clays, henna, fenugreek and more proven to increase the health of your hair. Try adding some of these to your routine. Opt for organic and research how to use them effectively.

Conditioning – The curlier your hair is the more important it is to condition, especially deep condition your hair. The use of a steamer or a hooded dryer with a shower cap can nourish, increase the elasticity, strength, shine and over health of your hair.

Detangling – Starting with finger detangling or a wide tooth comb reduces stress on the hair shaft, you can work down to a Denman brush once hair is thoroughly detangled to smooth strands. As hair is delicate, start detangling from the ends to the roots.

Hands – It is so tempting to play with the hair around your hairline or to twirl your ends. STOP! This is very damaging and will fray and break your hair.

Heat – Heat can be beneficial when conditioning your hair although should be avoided in other situations. Opt for indirect heat such as hooded dryers or no contact blow drying and never dry your hair until it is bone dry. When straightening, doing a roller set or flexi rod set before hand can reduce the amount of flat iron passes required. Always use a good quality heat protectant.

Massaging – Adding this to your hair regime isn't just for relaxation but also improves thickness and encourages hair growth. You can use scalp massagers or simply use your finger pads.

Moisturize and Hydrate – Hair needs water, it can be likened to flowers which start to wilt when it isn't getting enough. Keep on top of your moisturizing by regular inspecting your hair and scalp, spraying with a water and oil mix. If you wear your hair loose often, more moisture will be needed.

TIPS

Natural Oils and Butters – Adding these to your routine helps you to seal moisture into your hair and will promote stronger, longer and increased hair elasticity. Different oils and butters have different benefits so research is key!

Protective Styling – Hair retains more moisture in a protective style. Braids, twists and wigs will protect hair from daily stresses and help retain length. Ensure that your hair is clean, conditioned, moisturized and sealed well before installing. Winter is a good time to protect your hair as it can become brittle during this season. Avoid blow drying before installation and leaving in for more than 6 weeks. Give your hair a rest between protective styles and opt for looser styles to reduce stress to your scalp and edges.

Protein – Protein helps strengthen weak sections of the hair shaft and works best for porous hair. For protein sensitive hair, gentler treatments can prevent the hair from getting hard and brittle. Food will always be the best source of protein and way to get stronger hair (patience is required), however, there are fantastic products on the market which strengthen hair with the results being seen immediately. A combination of the two works best.

Retention – A good way to see if you have healthy hair is whether you can retain length. If your hair is breaking, inspect the state of your hair. Does it feel dry, spongy or brittle? Are your ends wispy, knotted, or split? Depending on its condition, it may need more moisture, protein, a change in your diet, a protective style or simply a good clarifying shampoo. Regularly monitoring your hair's health can help it to grow healthy and strong.

Shampooing – You may not need to shampoo every wash day - you can condition (co-wash) to cleanse and hydrate your hair between shampooing sessions. You also may not need to use a clarifying shampoo each time, depending on the products you use regularly.

TIPS

Shampooing (cont) – Have a couple of different types and switch them based on whether your hair needs a deep or light cleanse.

Stretching Styles – To get the most out of your hair, learning how to stretch (maintain while keeping healthy) styles over an extended period of time is vital! It reduces hair manipulation, damage, and gives you the flexibility to enjoy your hair to the fullest. Styles include blow outs, flat irons, chemical processing such as dyes and perms.

Supplements – It can be difficult to eat the perfect diet which targets both the hair and scalp. Good quality supplements will give our bodies the boost and nourishment it needs so that our hair can flourish. Supplements including biotin, folic acid and vitamin C work well with A, B and E vitamins being a bonus. Vitamin D, zinc and iron are also crucial in your diet. Beware as some supplements contain potent ingredients which may cause your hair to appear thicker temporarily however, when you stop using them, your hair quickly reverts back to its original condition.

Trimming and Cutting – The ends of your hair should be regularly inspected. Your hair won't grow well if you have unhealthy and damaged ends. You can routinely do a full trim or cut, but there will be times when your hair doesn't need it. Between cuts and trims, 'dust' your ends by removing damaged sections of individual hair strands.

On average, hair grows half an inch per month and learning how to retain this length is very important. Ultimately eating well and keeping hydrated (body and hair) will do the best for your hair in the long term. Keeping your hair routine simple, especially at first is the best way to gather information about your hair and find out which products and techniques work to bring the best out of it.

Invest in your hair, it is the crown you never take off

Hair Profile

Date: _____

Circle all that apply (refer to the **definitions** if needed):

Hair Type: 1 | 2 | 3 | 4 *and* a | b | c

Other: _____

Hair Thickness: Fine | Thin | Thick | Coarse

Hair Density: Low | Medium | High

Hair Porosity: Low | Medium | High

Overall Condition: Healthy | Damaged | Shiny | Dull | Soft
Dry | Brittle | Spongy | Rough | Smooth | Frizzy | _____

My Ends are: Split | Knotted | Wispy | Not sure

My Hair is: Natural (loose) | Locs | Relaxed | Texturized
Bleached | Dyed (non-bleach) | Other: _____

Last Cut: _____   **Last Trim:** _____

How would you describe your hair? _____
_____

Starting Hair Length (inches):

Top: _____   Crown: _____   Nape: _____

Above Ear (Left): _____   Above Ear (Right): _____

Below Ear (Left): _____   Below Ear (Right): _____

Problem Areas: (e.g. hairline, nape, dry, brittle, thin)

Hair Profile Continued...

How often do you:

	Daily	Twice Weekly	Weekly	Twice Monthly	Monthly	Less
Shampoo						
Condition						
Deep Condition						
Moisturize						
Blow Dry						
Flat Iron						
Trim						
Cut						
Protective Style						
Other						

How do you tend to style your hair? _____

_____

Comments: _____

_____

Hair Goals:

Daily Hair Tracker

Date: _____

	J	F	M	A	M	J	J	A	S	O	N	D	LEGEND
1													
2													☐
3													
4													☐
5													
6													☐
7													
8													☐
9													
10													☐
11													
12													☐
13													
14													☐
15													
16													☐
17													
18													☐
19													
20													☐
21													
22													☐
23													
24													☐
25													
26													☐
27													
28													☐
29													
30													☐
31													

Daily Hair Tracker

Date: _____

	J	F	M	A	M	J	J	A	S	O	N	D
1												
2												
3												
4												
5												
6												
7												
8												
9												
10												
11												
12												
13												
14												
15												
16												
17												
18												
19												
20												
21												
22												
23												
24												
25												
26												
27												
28												
29												
30												
31												

LEGEND

Wash Day

Date: _____

Reason for washing: Routine | Dry | Product Build Up

Other: _____

Home | Salon/Stylist: _____

Wet Process

	Product(s) / Tool(s) Used	Method(s) Used
Shampoo		
Conditioner		
Treatments		
Other		

Dry Process

Detangling		
Drying		
Styling		
Other		

Comments

_____

_____

_____

_____

Wash Day – The Process

The key is in the detail: Explain which products were used and their order. Include how your hair felt/reacted to the products, tools and methods used.

1. _____
2. _____
3. _____
4. _____
5. _____
6. _____
7. _____
8. _____
9. _____
10. _____
11. _____
12. _____
13. _____
14. _____
15. _____

What was the intention for your hair?

_____
_____

How did it turn out based on this expectation?

_____
_____

Learning points for next time:

My Hair:
Looks: /10
Feels: /10

Wash Day

Date: _____

Reason for washing: Routine | Dry | Product Build Up

Other: _____

Home | Salon/Stylist: _____

Wet Process

	Product(s) / Tool(s) Used	Method(s) Used
Shampoo		
Conditioner		
Treatments		
Other		

Dry Process

Detangling		
Drying		
Styling		
Other		

Comments

_____

_____

_____

_____

Wash Day – The Process

The key is in the detail: Explain which products were used and their order. Include how your hair felt/reacted to the products, tools and methods used.

1. _____
2. _____
3. _____
4. _____
5. _____
6. _____
7. _____
8. _____
9. _____
10. _____
11. _____
12. _____
13. _____
14. _____
15. _____

What was the intention for your hair?

_____
_____

How did it turn out based on this expectation?

_____
_____

Learning points for next time:

My Hair:
Looks: /10
Feels: /10

Wash Day

Date: _____

Reason for washing: Routine | Dry | Product Build Up

Other: _____

Home | Salon/Stylist: _____

Wet Process

	Product(s) / Tool(s) Used	Method(s) Used
Shampoo		
Conditioner		
Treatments		
Other		

Dry Process

Detangling		
Drying		
Styling		
Other		

Comments

_____

_____

_____

_____

wash Day – The Process

The key is in the detail: Explain which products were used and their order. Include how your hair felt/reacted to the products, tools and methods used.

1. _____
2. _____
3. _____
4. _____
5. _____
6. _____
7. _____
8. _____
9. _____
10. _____
11. _____
12. _____
13. _____
14. _____
15. _____

What was the intention for your hair?

_____
_____

How did it turn out based on this expectation?

_____
_____

Learning points for next time:

My Hair:
Looks: /10
Feels: /10

Wash Day

Date: _____

Reason for washing: Routine | Dry | Product Build Up

Other: _____

Home | Salon/Stylist: _____

Wet Process

	Product(s) / Tool(s) Used	Method(s) Used
Shampoo		
Conditioner		
Treatments		
Other		

Dry Process

Detangling		
Drying		
Styling		
Other		

Comments

_____

_____

_____

_____

Wash Day – The Process

The key is in the detail: Explain which products were used and their order. Include how your hair felt/reacted to the products, tools and methods used.

1. _____
2. _____
3. _____
4. _____
5. _____
6. _____
7. _____
8. _____
9. _____
10. _____
11. _____
12. _____
13. _____
14. _____
15. _____

What was the intention for your hair?

_____
_____

How did it turn out based on this expectation?

_____
_____

Learning points for next time:

My Hair:
Looks: /10
Feels: /10

Wash Day

Date: _____

Reason for washing: Routine | Dry | Product Build Up

Other: _____

Home | Salon/Stylist: _____

Wet Process

	Product(s) / Tool(s) Used	Method(s) Used
Shampoo		
Conditioner		
Treatments		
Other		

Dry Process

Detangling		
Drying		
Styling		
Other		

Comments

_____

_____

_____

_____

Wash Day – The Process

The key is in the detail: Explain which products were used and their order. Include how your hair felt/reacted to the products, tools and methods used.

1. _____
2. _____
3. _____
4. _____
5. _____
6. _____
7. _____
8. _____
9. _____
10. _____
11. _____
12. _____
13. _____
14. _____
15. _____

What was the intention for your hair?

_____
_____

How did it turn out based on this expectation?

_____
_____

Learning points for next time:

My Hair:
Looks: /10
Feels: /10

wash Day

Date: _____

Reason for washing: Routine | Dry | Product Build Up

Other: _____

Home | Salon/Stylist: _____

Wet Process

	Product(s) / Tool(s) Used	Method(s) Used
Shampoo		
Conditioner		
Treatments		
Other		

Dry Process

Detangling		
Drying		
Styling		
Other		

Comments

_____

_____

_____

_____

Wash Day – The Process

The key is in the detail: Explain which products were used and their order. Include how your hair felt/reacted to the products, tools and methods used.

1. _____
2. _____
3. _____
4. _____
5. _____
6. _____
7. _____
8. _____
9. _____
10. _____
11. _____
12. _____
13. _____
14. _____
15. _____

What was the intention for your hair?

_____
_____

How did it turn out based on this expectation?

_____
_____

Learning points for next time:

My Hair:
Looks: /10
Feels: /10

Wash Day

Date: _____

Reason for washing: Routine | Dry | Product Build Up

Other: _____

Home | Salon/Stylist: _____

Wet Process

	Product(s) / Tool(s) Used	Method(s) Used
Shampoo		
Conditioner		
Treatments		
Other		

Dry Process

Detangling		
Drying		
Styling		
Other		

Comments

_____
_____
_____
_____

Wash Day – The Process

The key is in the detail: Explain which products were used and their order. Include how your hair felt/reacted to the products, tools and methods used.

1. _____
2. _____
3. _____
4. _____
5. _____
6. _____
7. _____
8. _____
9. _____
10. _____
11. _____
12. _____
13. _____
14. _____
15. _____

What was the intention for your hair?

_____

_____

How did it turn out based on this expectation?

_____

_____

Learning points for next time:

My Hair:
Looks: /10
Feels: /10

Wash Day

Date: _____

Reason for washing: Routine | Dry | Product Build Up

Other: _____

Home | Salon/Stylist: _____

Wet Process

	Product(s) / Tool(s) Used	Method(s) Used
Shampoo		
Conditioner		
Treatments		
Other		

Dry Process

Detangling		
Drying		
Styling		
Other		

Comments

_____

_____

_____

_____

Wash Day – The Process

The key is in the detail: Explain which products were used and their order. Include how your hair felt/reacted to the products, tools and methods used.

1. _____
2. _____
3. _____
4. _____
5. _____
6. _____
7. _____
8. _____
9. _____
10. _____
11. _____
12. _____
13. _____
14. _____
15. _____

What was the intention for your hair?

_____

_____

How did it turn out based on this expectation?

_____

_____

Learning points for next time:

My Hair:
Looks: /10
Feels: /10

Wash Day

Date: _____

Reason for washing: Routine | Dry | Product Build Up

Other: _____

Home | Salon/Stylist: _____

Wet Process

	Product(s) / Tool(s) Used	Method(s) Used
Shampoo		
Conditioner		
Treatments		
Other		

Dry Process

Detangling		
Drying		
Styling		
Other		

Comments

_____

_____

_____

_____

Wash Day – The Process

The key is in the detail: Explain which products were used and their order. Include how your hair felt/reacted to the products, tools and methods used.

1. _____
2. _____
3. _____
4. _____
5. _____
6. _____
7. _____
8. _____
9. _____
10. _____
11. _____
12. _____
13. _____
14. _____
15. _____

What was the intention for your hair?

_____
_____

How did it turn out based on this expectation?

_____
_____

Learning points for next time:

My Hair:
Looks: /10
Feels: /10

Wash Day

Date: _____

Reason for washing: Routine | Dry | Product Build Up

Other: _____

Home | Salon/Stylist: _____

Wet Process

	Product(s) / Tool(s) Used	Method(s) Used
Shampoo		
Conditioner		
Treatments		
Other		

Dry Process

Detangling		
Drying		
Styling		
Other		

Comments

_____

_____

_____

_____

Wash Day – The Process

The key is in the detail: Explain which products were used and their order. Include how your hair felt/reacted to the products, tools and methods used.

1. _____
2. _____
3. _____
4. _____
5. _____
6. _____
7. _____
8. _____
9. _____
10. _____
11. _____
12. _____
13. _____
14. _____
15. _____

What was the intention for your hair?

_____

_____

How did it turn out based on this expectation?

_____

_____

Learning points for next time:

My Hair:
Looks: /10
Feels: /10

WASH DAY

Date: _____

Reason for washing: Routine | Dry | Product Build Up

Other: _____

Home | Salon/Stylist: _____

Wet Process

	Product(s) / Tool(s) Used	Method(s) Used
Shampoo		
Conditioner		
Treatments		
Other		

Dry Process

Detangling		
Drying		
Styling		
Other		

Comments

_____

_____

_____

_____

Wash Day – The Process

The key is in the detail: Explain which products were used and their order. Include how your hair felt/reacted to the products, tools and methods used.

1. _____
2. _____
3. _____
4. _____
5. _____
6. _____
7. _____
8. _____
9. _____
10. _____
11. _____
12. _____
13. _____
14. _____
15. _____

What was the intention for your hair?

_____

_____

How did it turn out based on this expectation?

_____

_____

Learning points for next time:

My Hair:
Looks: /10
Feels: /10

Wash Day

Date: _____

Reason for washing: Routine | Dry | Product Build Up

Other: _____

Home | Salon/Stylist: _____

Wet Process

	Product(s) / Tool(s) Used	Method(s) Used
Shampoo		
Conditioner		
Treatments		
Other		

Dry Process

Detangling		
Drying		
Styling		
Other		

Comments

_____

_____

_____

_____

Wash Day – The Process

The key is in the detail: Explain which products were used and their order. Include how your hair felt/reacted to the products, tools and methods used.

1. _____
2. _____
3. _____
4. _____
5. _____
6. _____
7. _____
8. _____
9. _____
10. _____
11. _____
12. _____
13. _____
14. _____
15. _____

What was the intention for your hair?

_____
_____

How did it turn out based on this expectation?

_____
_____

Learning points for next time:

My Hair:
Looks: /10
Feels: /10

Wash Day

Date: _____

Reason for washing: Routine | Dry | Product Build Up

Other: _____

Home | Salon/Stylist: _____

Wet Process

	Product(s) / Tool(s) Used	Method(s) Used
Shampoo		
Conditioner		
Treatments		
Other		

Dry Process

Detangling		
Drying		
Styling		
Other		

Comments

_____

_____

_____

_____

Wash Day – The Process

The key is in the detail: Explain which products were used and their order. Include how your hair felt/reacted to the products, tools and methods used.

1. _____
2. _____
3. _____
4. _____
5. _____
6. _____
7. _____
8. _____
9. _____
10. _____
11. _____
12. _____
13. _____
14. _____
15. _____

What was the intention for your hair?

_____
_____

How did it turn out based on this expectation?

_____
_____

Learning points for next time:

My Hair:
Looks: /10
Feels: /10

Time to Switch it up!

Your hair can benefit when you shake things up a little bit!

Try adding another oil to your routine! Oils can be deeply nourishing for hair and different oils have a host of different benefits! You can add oils before you shampoo, with your conditioner, or as part of your style prep!

*When using some oils, you may get immediate results, however, with most natural products, you will need to use it a few times in order to see a noticeable change. Patience will serve you well.

What oil(s) did you add to your hair routine and how?

_____

_____

_____

What are the hair benefits of this oil?

_____

_____

_____

Did you notice any changes with your hair?*

_____

_____

_____

_____

Notes

Wash Day

Date: _____

Reason for washing: Routine | Dry | Product Build Up

Other: _____

Home | Salon/Stylist: _____

Wet Process

	Product(s) / Tool(s) Used	Method(s) Used
Shampoo		
Conditioner		
Treatments		
Other		

Dry Process

Detangling		
Drying		
Styling		
Other		

Comments

_____

_____

_____

_____

Wash Day – The Process

The key is in the detail: Explain which products were used and their order. Include how your hair felt/reacted to the products, tools and methods used.

1. _____
2. _____
3. _____
4. _____
5. _____
6. _____
7. _____
8. _____
9. _____
10. _____
11. _____
12. _____
13. _____
14. _____
15. _____

What was the intention for your hair?

_____

_____

How did it turn out based on this expectation?

_____

_____

Learning points for next time:

My Hair:
Looks: /10
Feels: /10

Wash Day

Date: _____

Reason for washing: Routine | Dry | Product Build Up

Other: _____

Home | Salon/Stylist: _____

Wet Process

	Product(s) / Tool(s) Used	Method(s) Used
Shampoo		
Conditioner		
Treatments		
Other		

Dry Process

Detangling		
Drying		
Styling		
Other		

Comments

_____

_____

_____

_____

Wash Day – The Process

The key is in the detail: Explain which products were used and their order. Include how your hair felt/reacted to the products, tools and methods used.

1. _____
2. _____
3. _____
4. _____
5. _____
6. _____
7. _____
8. _____
9. _____
10. _____
11. _____
12. _____
13. _____
14. _____
15. _____

What was the intention for your hair?

_____

_____

How did it turn out based on this expectation?

_____

_____

Learning points for next time:

My Hair:
Looks: /10
Feels: /10

Wash Day

Date: _____

Reason for washing: Routine | Dry | Product Build Up

Other: _____

Home | Salon/Stylist: _____

Wet Process

	Product(s) / Tool(s) Used	Method(s) Used
Shampoo		
Conditioner		
Treatments		
Other		

Dry Process

Detangling		
Drying		
Styling		
Other		

Comments

_____

_____

_____

_____

Wash Day – The Process

The key is in the detail: Explain which products were used and their order. Include how your hair felt/reacted to the products, tools and methods used.

1. _____
2. _____
3. _____
4. _____
5. _____
6. _____
7. _____
8. _____
9. _____
10. _____
11. _____
12. _____
13. _____
14. _____
15. _____

What was the intention for your hair?

_____
_____

How did it turn out based on this expectation?

_____
_____

Learning points for next time:

My Hair:
Looks: /10
Feels: /10

Wash Day

Date: _____

Reason for washing: Routine | Dry | Product Build Up

Other: _____

Home | Salon/Stylist: _____

Wet Process

	Product(s) / Tool(s) Used	Method(s) Used
Shampoo		
Conditioner		
Treatments		
Other		

Dry Process

Detangling		
Drying		
Styling		
Other		

Comments

_____

_____

_____

_____

Wash Day – The Process

The key is in the detail: Explain which products were used and their order. Include how your hair felt/reacted to the products, tools and methods used.

1. _____
2. _____
3. _____
4. _____
5. _____
6. _____
7. _____
8. _____
9. _____
10. _____
11. _____
12. _____
13. _____
14. _____
15. _____

What was the intention for your hair?

_____
_____

How did it turn out based on this expectation?

_____
_____

Learning points for next time:

My Hair:
Looks: /10
Feels: /10

Wash Day

Date: _____

Reason for washing: Routine | Dry | Product Build Up

Other: _____

Home | Salon/Stylist: _____

Wet Process

	Product(s) / Tool(s) Used	Method(s) Used
Shampoo		
Conditioner		
Treatments		
Other		

Dry Process

Detangling		
Drying		
Styling		
Other		

Comments

_____

_____

_____

_____

Wash Day – The Process

The key is in the detail: Explain which products were used and their order. Include how your hair felt/reacted to the products, tools and methods used.

1. _____
2. _____
3. _____
4. _____
5. _____
6. _____
7. _____
8. _____
9. _____
10. _____
11. _____
12. _____
13. _____
14. _____
15. _____

What was the intention for your hair?

_____
_____

How did it turn out based on this expectation?

_____
_____

Learning points for next time:

My Hair:
Looks: /10
Feels: /10

Wash Day

Date: _____

Reason for washing: Routine | Dry | Product Build Up

Other: _____

Home | Salon/Stylist: _____

Wet Process

	Product(s) / Tool(s) Used	Method(s) Used
Shampoo		
Conditioner		
Treatments		
Other		

Dry Process

Detangling		
Drying		
Styling		
Other		

Comments

_____

_____

_____

_____

Wash Day – The Process

The key is in the detail: Explain which products were used and their order. Include how your hair felt/reacted to the products, tools and methods used.

1. _____
2. _____
3. _____
4. _____
5. _____
6. _____
7. _____
8. _____
9. _____
10. _____
11. _____
12. _____
13. _____
14. _____
15. _____

What was the intention for your hair?

_____
_____

How did it turn out based on this expectation?

_____
_____

Learning points for next time:

My Hair:
Looks: /10
Feels: /10

Wash Day

Date: _____

Reason for washing: Routine | Dry | Product Build Up

Other: _____

Home | Salon/Stylist: _____

Wet Process

	Product(s) / Tool(s) Used	Method(s) Used
Shampoo		
Conditioner		
Treatments		
Other		

Dry Process

Detangling		
Drying		
Styling		
Other		

Comments

_____

_____

_____

_____

Wash Day – The Process

The key is in the detail: Explain which products were used and their order. Include how your hair felt/reacted to the products, tools and methods used.

1. _____
2. _____
3. _____
4. _____
5. _____
6. _____
7. _____
8. _____
9. _____
10. _____
11. _____
12. _____
13. _____
14. _____
15. _____

What was the intention for your hair?

_____
_____

How did it turn out based on this expectation?

_____
_____

Learning points for next time:

My Hair:
Looks: /10
Feels: /10

Wash Day

Date: _____

Reason for washing: Routine | Dry | Product Build Up

Other: _____

Home | Salon/Stylist: _____

Wet Process

	Product(s) / Tool(s) Used	Method(s) Used
Shampoo		
Conditioner		
Treatments		
Other		

Dry Process

Detangling		
Drying		
Styling		
Other		

Comments

_____

_____

_____

_____

Wash Day – The Process

The key is in the detail: Explain which products were used and their order. Include how your hair felt/reacted to the products, tools and methods used.

1. _____
2. _____
3. _____
4. _____
5. _____
6. _____
7. _____
8. _____
9. _____
10. _____
11. _____
12. _____
13. _____
14. _____
15. _____

What was the intention for your hair?

_____
_____

How did it turn out based on this expectation?

_____
_____

Learning points for next time:

My Hair:
Looks: /10
Feels: /10

Wash Day

Date: _____

Reason for washing: Routine | Dry | Product Build Up

Other: _____

Home | Salon/Stylist: _____

Wet Process

	Product(s) / Tool(s) Used	Method(s) Used
Shampoo		
Conditioner		
Treatments		
Other		

Dry Process

Detangling		
Drying		
Styling		
Other		

Comments

_____

_____

_____

_____

Wash Day – The Process

The key is in the detail: Explain which products were used and their order. Include how your hair felt/reacted to the products, tools and methods used.

1. _____
2. _____
3. _____
4. _____
5. _____
6. _____
7. _____
8. _____
9. _____
10. _____
11. _____
12. _____
13. _____
14. _____
15. _____

What was the intention for your hair?

_____
_____

How did it turn out based on this expectation?

_____
_____

Learning points for next time:

My Hair:
Looks: /10
Feels: /10

Wash Day

Date: _____

Reason for washing: Routine | Dry | Product Build Up

Other: _____

Home | Salon/Stylist: _____

Wet Process

	Product(s) / Tool(s) Used	Method(s) Used
Shampoo		
Conditioner		
Treatments		
Other		

Dry Process

Detangling		
Drying		
Styling		
Other		

Comments

_____

_____

_____

_____

Wash Day – The Process

The key is in the detail: Explain which products were used and their order. Include how your hair felt/reacted to the products, tools and methods used.

1. _____
2. _____
3. _____
4. _____
5. _____
6. _____
7. _____
8. _____
9. _____
10. _____
11. _____
12. _____
13. _____
14. _____
15. _____

What was the intention for your hair?

_____
_____

How did it turn out based on this expectation?

_____
_____

Learning points for next time:

My Hair:
Looks: /10
Feels: /10

Time to Switch it Up!

Your hair can benefit when you shake things up a little bit!

Try adding a natural cleanser such as a clay, or treatment to your routine! The natural herbs used in Ayurvedic hair recipes can work wonders by increasing shine, thickening, strengthening your hair and more! It can be a messy process and difficult to use, especially at first, however mix with your shampoo or conditioner before going neat!

*When using natural remedies, you may need to use them a few times in order to see a noticeable change.

What natural recipes did you use and how?

_____
_____
_____

What are the hair benefits of the ingredients?

_____
_____
_____

Did you notice any changes with your hair?*

_____
_____
_____
_____

Notes

Wash Day

Date: _____

Reason for washing: Routine | Dry | Product Build Up

Other: _____

Home | Salon/Stylist: _____

Wet Process

	Product(s) / Tool(s) Used	Method(s) Used
Shampoo		
Conditioner		
Treatments		
Other		

Dry Process

Detangling		
Drying		
Styling		
Other		

Comments

_____

_____

_____

_____

Wash Day – The Process

The key is in the detail: Explain which products were used and their order. Include how your hair felt/reacted to the products, tools and methods used.

1. _____
2. _____
3. _____
4. _____
5. _____
6. _____
7. _____
8. _____
9. _____
10. _____
11. _____
12. _____
13. _____
14. _____
15. _____

What was the intention for your hair?

_____
_____

How did it turn out based on this expectation?

_____
_____

Learning points for next time:

My Hair:
Looks: /10
Feels: /10

Wash Day

Date: _____

Reason for washing: Routine | Dry | Product Build Up

Other: _____

Home | Salon/Stylist: _____

Wet Process

	Product(s) / Tool(s) Used	Method(s) Used
Shampoo		
Conditioner		
Treatments		
Other		

Dry Process

Detangling		
Drying		
Styling		
Other		

Comments

_____

_____

_____

_____

Wash Day – The Process

The key is in the detail: Explain which products were used and their order. Include how your hair felt/reacted to the products, tools and methods used.

1. _____
2. _____
3. _____
4. _____
5. _____
6. _____
7. _____
8. _____
9. _____
10. _____
11. _____
12. _____
13. _____
14. _____
15. _____

What was the intention for your hair?

_____

_____

How did it turn out based on this expectation?

_____

_____

Learning points for next time:

My Hair:
Looks: /10
Feels: /10

Wash Day

Date: _____

Reason for washing: Routine | Dry | Product Build Up

Other: _____

Home | Salon/Stylist: _____

Wet Process

	Product(s) / Tool(s) Used	Method(s) Used
Shampoo		
Conditioner		
Treatments		
Other		

Dry Process

Detangling		
Drying		
Styling		
Other		

Comments

_____

_____

_____

_____

Wash Day – The Process

The key is in the detail: Explain which products were used and their order. Include how your hair felt/reacted to the products, tools and methods used.

1. _____
2. _____
3. _____
4. _____
5. _____
6. _____
7. _____
8. _____
9. _____
10. _____
11. _____
12. _____
13. _____
14. _____
15. _____

What was the intention for your hair?

_____
_____

How did it turn out based on this expectation?

_____
_____

Learning points for next time:

My Hair:
Looks: /10
Feels: /10

Wash Day

Date: _____

Reason for washing: Routine | Dry | Product Build Up

Other: _____

Home | Salon/Stylist: _____

Wet Process

	Product(s) / Tool(s) Used	Method(s) Used
Shampoo		
Conditioner		
Treatments		
Other		

Dry Process

Detangling		
Drying		
Styling		
Other		

Comments

_____

_____

_____

_____

Wash Day – The Process

The key is in the detail: Explain which products were used and their order. Include how your hair felt/reacted to the products, too s and methods used.

1. _____
2. _____
3. _____
4. _____
5. _____
6. _____
7. _____
8. _____
9. _____
10. _____
11. _____
12. _____
13. _____
14. _____
15. _____

What was the intention for your hair?

_____
_____

How did it turn out based on this expectation?

_____
_____

Learning points for next time:

My Hair:
Looks: /10
Feels: /10

Wash Day

Date: _____

Reason for washing: Routine | Dry | Product Build Up

Other: _____

Home | Salon/Stylist: _____

Wet Process

	Product(s) / Tool(s) Used	Method(s) Used
Shampoo		
Conditioner		
Treatments		
Other		

Dry Process

Detangling		
Drying		
Styling		
Other		

Comments

_____

_____

_____

_____

Wash Day – The Process

The key is in the detail: Explain which products were used and their order. Include how your hair felt/reacted to the products, tools and methods used.

1. _____
2. _____
3. _____
4. _____
5. _____
6. _____
7. _____
8. _____
9. _____
10. _____
11. _____
12. _____
13. _____
14. _____
15. _____

What was the intention for your hair?

_____

_____

How did it turn out based on this expectation?

_____

_____

Learning points for next time:

My Hair:
Looks: /10
Feels: /10

Wash Day

Date: _____

Reason for washing: Routine | Dry | Product Build Up

Other: _____

Home | Salon/Stylist: _____

Wet Process

	Product(s) / Tool(s) Used	Method(s) Used
Shampoo		
Conditioner		
Treatments		
Other		

Dry Process

Detangling		
Drying		
Styling		
Other		

Comments

_____

_____

_____

_____

Wash Day – The Process

The key is in the detail: Explain which products were used and their order. Include how your hair felt/reacted to the products, tools and methods used.

1. _____
2. _____
3. _____
4. _____
5. _____
6. _____
7. _____
8. _____
9. _____
10. _____
11. _____
12. _____
13. _____
14. _____
15. _____

What was the intention for your hair?

_____

_____

How did it turn out based on this expectation?

_____

_____

Learning points for next time:

My Hair:
Looks: /10
Feels: /10

Wash Day   Date: _____

Reason for washing: Routine | Dry | Product Build Up

Other: _____

Home | Salon/Stylist: _____

Wet Process

	Product(s) / Tool(s) Used	Method(s) Used
Shampoo		
Conditioner		
Treatments		
Other		

Dry Process

Detangling		
Drying		
Styling		
Other		

Comments

_____

_____

_____

_____

Wash Day – The Process

The key is in the detail: Explain which products were used and their order. Include how your hair felt/reacted to the products, tools and methods used.

1. _____
2. _____
3. _____
4. _____
5. _____
6. _____
7. _____
8. _____
9. _____
10. _____
11. _____
12. _____
13. _____
14. _____
15. _____

What was the intention for your hair?

_____
_____

How did it turn out based on this expectation?

_____
_____

Learning points for next time:

My Hair:
Looks: /10
Feels: /10

Wash Day

Date: _____

Reason for washing: Routine | Dry | Product Build Up

Other: _____

Home | Salon/Stylist: _____

Wet Process

	Product(s) / Tool(s) Used	Method(s) Used
Shampoo		
Conditioner		
Treatments		
Other		

Dry Process

Detangling		
Drying		
Styling		
Other		

Comments

_____

_____

_____

_____

Wash Day – The Process

The key is in the detail: Explain which products were used and their order. Include how your hair felt/reacted to the products, tools and methods used.

1. _____
2. _____
3. _____
4. _____
5. _____
6. _____
7. _____
8. _____
9. _____
10. _____
11. _____
12. _____
13. _____
14. _____
15. _____

What was the intention for your hair?

_____
_____

How did it turn out based on this expectation?

_____
_____

Learning points for next time:

My Hair:
Looks: /10
Feels: /10

Wash Day

Date: _____

Reason for washing: Routine | Dry | Product Build Up

Other: _____

Home | Salon/Stylist: _____

Wet Process

	Product(s) / Tool(s) Used	Method(s) Used
Shampoo		
Conditioner		
Treatments		
Other		

Dry Process

Detangling		
Drying		
Styling		
Other		

Comments

_____

_____

_____

_____

Wash Day – The Process

The key is in the detail: Explain which products were used and their order. Include how your hair felt/reacted to the products, tools and methods used.

1. _____
2. _____
3. _____
4. _____
5. _____
6. _____
7. _____
8. _____
9. _____
10. _____
11. _____
12. _____
13. _____
14. _____
15. _____

What was the intention for your hair?

_____

_____

How did it turn out based on this expectation?

_____

_____

Learning points for next time:

My Hair:
Looks: /10
Feels: /10

Wash Day

Date: _____

Reason for washing: Routine | Dry | Product Build Up

Other: _____

Home | Salon/Stylist: _____

Wet Process

	Product(s) / Tool(s) Used	Method(s) Used
Shampoo		
Conditioner		
Treatments		
Other		

Dry Process

Detangling		
Drying		
Styling		
Other		

Comments

_____

_____

_____

_____

Wash Day – The Process

The key is in the detail: Explain which products were used and their order. Include how your hair felt/reacted to the products, tools and methods used.

1. _____
2. _____
3. _____
4. _____
5. _____
6. _____
7. _____
8. _____
9. _____
10. _____
11. _____
12. _____
13. _____
14. _____
15. _____

What was the intention for your hair?

_____
_____

How did it turn out based on this expectation?

_____
_____

Learning points for next time:

My Hair:
Looks: /10
Feels: /10

Wash Day

Date: _____

Reason for washing: Routine | Dry | Product Build Up

Other: _____

Home | Salon/Stylist: _____

Wet Process

	Product(s) / Tool(s) Used	Method(s) Used
Shampoo		
Conditioner		
Treatments		
Other		

Dry Process

Detangling		
Drying		
Styling		
Other		

Comments

_____

_____

_____

_____

Wash Day – The Process

The key is in the detail: Explain which products were used and their order. Include how your hair felt/reacted to the products, tools and methods used.

1. _____
2. _____
3. _____
4. _____
5. _____
6. _____
7. _____
8. _____
9. _____
10. _____
11. _____
12. _____
13. _____
14. _____
15. _____

What was the intention for your hair?

_____

_____

How did it turn out based on this expectation?

_____

_____

Learning points for next time:

My Hair:
Looks: /10
Feels: /10

Wash Day

Date: _____

Reason for washing: Routine | Dry | Product Build Up

Other: _____

Home | Salon/Stylist: _____

Wet Process

	Product(s) / Tool(s) Used	Method(s) Used
Shampoo		
Conditioner		
Treatments		
Other		

Dry Process

Detangling		
Drying		
Styling		
Other		

Comments

_____

_____

_____

_____

Wash Day – The Process

The key is in the detail: Explain which products were used and their order. Include how your hair felt/reacted to the products, tools and methods used.

1. _____
2. _____
3. _____
4. _____
5. _____
6. _____
7. _____
8. _____
9. _____
10. _____
11. _____
12. _____
13. _____
14. _____
15. _____

What was the intention for your hair?

_____

_____

How did it turn out based on this expectation?

_____

_____

Learning points for next time:

My Hair:
Looks: /10
Feels: /10

Wash Day

Date: _____

Reason for washing: Routine | Dry | Product Build Up

Other: _____

Home | Salon/Stylist: _____

Wet Process

	Product(s) / Tool(s) Used	Method(s) Used
Shampoo		
Conditioner		
Treatments		
Other		

Dry Process

Detangling		
Drying		
Styling		
Other		

Comments

_____

_____

_____

_____

Wash Day – The Process

The key is in the detail: Explain which products were used and their order. Include how your hair felt/reacted to the products, tools and methods used.

1. _____
2. _____
3. _____
4. _____
5. _____
6. _____
7. _____
8. _____
9. _____
10. _____
11. _____
12. _____
13. _____
14. _____
15. _____

What was the intention for your hair?

_____
_____

How did it turn out based on this expectation?

_____
_____

Learning points for next time:

My Hair:
Looks: /10
Feels: /10

Wash Day

Date: _____

Reason for washing: Routine | Dry | Product Build Up

Other: _____

Home | Salon/Stylist: _____

Wet Process

	Product(s) / Tool(s) Used	Method(s) Used
Shampoo		
Conditioner		
Treatments		
Other		

Dry Process

Detangling		
Drying		
Styling		
Other		

Comments

_____

_____

_____

_____

Wash Day – The Process

The key is in the detail: Explain which products were used and their order. Include how your hair felt/reacted to the products, tools and methods used.

1. _____
2. _____
3. _____
4. _____
5. _____
6. _____
7. _____
8. _____
9. _____
10. _____
11. _____
12. _____
13. _____
14. _____
15. _____

What was the intention for your hair?

_____

_____

How did it turn out based on this expectation?

_____

_____

Learning points for next time:

My Hair:
Looks: /10
Feels: /10

Time to Switch it up!

Your hair can benefit when you shake things up a little bit!

Try adding scalp exfoliation and/or scalp massages to your routine. Massages increase blood flow to your hair follicles, stimulate growth and promotes a healthy scalp! Exfoliation has these benefits but also removes excess skin cells and oil. Exfoliation can be chemical or physical.

A scalp massager can be used when washing hair or just after conditioning. It is safe to massage your scalp daily, however, exfoliate your scalp no more than once weekly.

Did you use any of these techniques and why?

_____

_____

_____

If yes, how did you use them in your routine?

_____

_____

_____

Did you notice any changes with your hair or scalp?

_____

_____

_____

Notes

Wash Day

Date: _____

Reason for washing: Routine | Dry | Product Build Up

Other: _____

Home | Salon/Stylist: _____

Wet Process

	Product(s) / Tool(s) Used	Method(s) Used
Shampoo		
Conditioner		
Treatments		
Other		

Dry Process

Detangling		
Drying		
Styling		
Other		

Comments

_____

_____

_____

_____

Wash Day – The Process

The key is in the detail: Explain which products were used and their order. Include how your hair felt/reacted to the products, tools and methods used.

1. _____
2. _____
3. _____
4. _____
5. _____
6. _____
7. _____
8. _____
9. _____
10. _____
11. _____
12. _____
13. _____
14. _____
15. _____

What was the intention for your hair?

_____
_____

How did it turn out based on this expectation?

_____
_____

Learning points for next time:

My Hair:
Looks: /10
Feels: /10

Wash Day

Date: _____

Reason for washing: Routine | Dry | Product Build Up

Other: _____

Home | Salon/Stylist: _____

Wet Process

	Product(s) / Tool(s) Used	Method(s) Used
Shampoo		
Conditioner		
Treatments		
Other		

Dry Process

Detangling		
Drying		
Styling		
Other		

Comments

_____

_____

_____

_____

Wash Day – The Process

The key is in the detail: Explain which products were used and their order. Include how your hair felt/reacted to the products, tools and methods used.

1. _____
2. _____
3. _____
4. _____
5. _____
6. _____
7. _____
8. _____
9. _____
10. _____
11. _____
12. _____
13. _____
14. _____
15. _____

What was the intention for your hair?

_____

_____

How did it turn out based on this expectation?

_____

_____

Learning points for next time:

My Hair:
Looks: /10
Feels: /10

Wash Day

Date: _____

Reason for washing: Routine | Dry | Product Build Up

Other: _____

Home | Salon/Stylist: _____

Wet Process

	Product(s) / Tool(s) Used	Method(s) Used
Shampoo		
Conditioner		
Treatments		
Other		

Dry Process

Detangling		
Drying		
Styling		
Other		

Comments

_____

_____

_____

_____

Wash Day – The Process

The key is in the detail: Explain which products were used and their order. Include how your hair felt/reacted to the products, tools and methods used.

1. _____
2. _____
3. _____
4. _____
5. _____
6. _____
7. _____
8. _____
9. _____
10. _____
11. _____
12. _____
13. _____
14. _____
15. _____

What was the intention for your hair?

_____

_____

How did it turn out based on this expectation?

_____

_____

Learning points for next time:

My Hair:
Looks: /10
Feels: /10

Wash Day

Date: _____

Reason for washing: Routine | Dry | Product Build Up

Other: _____

Home | Salon/Stylist: _____

Wet Process

	Product(s) / Tool(s) Used	Method(s) Used
Shampoo		
Conditioner		
Treatments		
Other		

Dry Process

Detangling		
Drying		
Styling		
Other		

Comments

_____

_____

_____

_____

Wash Day – The Process

The key is in the detail: Explain which products were used and their order. Include how your hair felt/reacted to the products, tools and methods used.

1. _____
2. _____
3. _____
4. _____
5. _____
6. _____
7. _____
8. _____
9. _____
10. _____
11. _____
12. _____
13. _____
14. _____
15. _____

What was the intention for your hair?

_____

_____

How did it turn out based on this expectation?

_____

_____

Learning points for next time:

My Hair:
Looks: /10
Feels: /10

Wash Day

Date: _____

Reason for washing: Routine | Dry | Product Build Up

Other: _____

Home | Salon/Stylist: _____

Wet Process

	Product(s) / Tool(s) Used	Method(s) Used
Shampoo		
Conditioner		
Treatments		
Other		

Dry Process

Detangling		
Drying		
Styling		
Other		

Comments

_____

_____

_____

_____

Wash Day – The Process

The key is in the detail: Explain which products were used and their order. Include how your hair felt/reacted to the products, tools and methods used.

1. _____
2. _____
3. _____
4. _____
5. _____
6. _____
7. _____
8. _____
9. _____
10. _____
11. _____
12. _____
13. _____
14. _____
15. _____

What was the intention for your hair?

_____

_____

How did it turn out based on this expectation?

_____

_____

Learning points for next time:

My Hair:
Looks: /10
Feels: /10

Wash Day

Date: _____

Reason for washing: Routine | Dry | Product Build Up

Other: _____

Home | Salon/Stylist: _____

Wet Process

	Product(s) / Tool(s) Used	Method(s) Used
Shampoo		
Conditioner		
Treatments		
Other		

Dry Process

Detangling		
Drying		
Styling		
Other		

Comments

_____

_____

_____

_____

Wash Day – The Process

The key is in the detail: Explain which products were used and their order. Include how your hair felt/reacted to the products, tools and methods used.

1. _____
2. _____
3. _____
4. _____
5. _____
6. _____
7. _____
8. _____
9. _____
10. _____
11. _____
12. _____
13. _____
14. _____
15. _____

What was the intention for your hair?

_____

_____

How did it turn out based on this expectation?

_____

_____

Learning points for next time:

My Hair:
Looks: /10
Feels: /10

Wash Day

Date: _____

Reason for washing: Routine | Dry | Product Build Up

Other: _____

Home | Salon/Stylist: _____

Wet Process

	Product(s) / Tool(s) Used	Method(s) Used
Shampoo		
Conditioner		
Treatments		
Other		

Dry Process

Detangling		
Drying		
Styling		
Other		

Comments

_____

_____

_____

_____

Wash Day – The Process

The key is in the detail: Explain which products were used and their order. Include how your hair felt/reacted to the products, tools and methods used.

1. _____
2. _____
3. _____
4. _____
5. _____
6. _____
7. _____
8. _____
9. _____
10. _____
11. _____
12. _____
13. _____
14. _____
15. _____

What was the intention for your hair?

_____

_____

How did it turn out based on this expectation?

_____

_____

Learning points for next time:

My Hair:
Looks: /10
Feels: /10

Wash Day   Date: _____

Reason for washing: Routine | Dry | Product Build Up

Other: _____

Home | Salon/Stylist: _____

Wet Process

	Product(s) / Tool(s) Used	Method(s) Used
Shampoo		
Conditioner		
Treatments		
Other		

Dry Process

Detangling		
Drying		
Styling		
Other		

Comments

_____

_____

_____

_____

Wash Day – The Process

The key is in the detail: Explain which products were used and their order. Include how your hair felt/reacted to the products, tools and methods used.

1. _____
2. _____
3. _____
4. _____
5. _____
6. _____
7. _____
8. _____
9. _____
10. _____
11. _____
12. _____
13. _____
14. _____
15. _____

What was the intention for your hair?

_____

_____

How did it turn out based on this expectation?

_____

_____

Learning points for next time:

My Hair:
Looks: /10
Feels: /10

Wash Day

Date: _____

Reason for washing: Routine | Dry | Product Build Up

Other: _____

Home | Salon/Stylist: _____

Wet Process

	Product(s) / Tool(s) Used	Method(s) Used
Shampoo		
Conditioner		
Treatments		
Other		

Dry Process

Detangling		
Drying		
Styling		
Other		

Comments

_____

_____

_____

_____

Wash Day – The Process

The key is in the detail: Explain which products were used and their order. Include how your hair felt/reacted to the products, tools and methods used.

1. _____
2. _____
3. _____
4. _____
5. _____
6. _____
7. _____
8. _____
9. _____
10. _____
11. _____
12. _____
13. _____
14. _____
15. _____

What was the intention for your hair?

_____
_____

How did it turn out based on this expectation?

_____
_____

Learning points for next time:

My Hair:
Looks: /10
Feels: /10

Wash Day

Date: _____

Reason for washing: Routine | Dry | Product Build Up

Other: _____

Home | Salon/Stylist: _____

Wet Process

	Product(s) / Tool(s) Used	Method(s) Used
Shampoo		
Conditioner		
Treatments		
Other		

Dry Process

Detangling		
Drying		
Styling		
Other		

Comments

_____

_____

_____

_____

Wash Day – The Process

The key is in the detail: Explain which products were used and their order. Include how your hair felt/reacted to the products, tools and methods used.

1. _____
2. _____
3. _____
4. _____
5. _____
6. _____
7. _____
8. _____
9. _____
10. _____
11. _____
12. _____
13. _____
14. _____
15. _____

What was the intention for your hair?

_____
_____

How did it turn out based on this expectation?

_____
_____

Learning points for next time:

My Hair:
Looks: /10
Feels: /10

Wash Day

Date: _____

Reason for washing: Routine | Dry | Product Build Up

Other: _____

Home | Salon/Stylist: _____

Wet Process

	Product(s) / Tool(s) Used	Method(s) Used
Shampoo		
Conditioner		
Treatments		
Other		

Dry Process

Detangling		
Drying		
Styling		
Other		

Comments

_____

_____

_____

_____

Wash Day – The Process

The key is in the detail: Explain which products were used and their order. Include how your hair felt/reacted to the products, tools and methods used.

1. _____
2. _____
3. _____
4. _____
5. _____
6. _____
7. _____
8. _____
9. _____
10. _____
11. _____
12. _____
13. _____
14. _____
15. _____

What was the intention for your hair?

_____

_____

How did it turn out based on this expectation?

_____

_____

Learning points for next time:

My Hair:
Looks: /10
Feels: /10

Wash Day

Date: _____

Reason for washing: Routine | Dry | Product Build Up

Other: _____

Home | Salon/Stylist: _____

Wet Process

	Product(s) / Tool(s) Used	Method(s) Used
Shampoo		
Conditioner		
Treatments		
Other		

Dry Process

Detangling		
Drying		
Styling		
Other		

Comments

_____

_____

_____

_____

Wash Day – The Process

The key is in the detail: Explain which products were used and their order. Include how your hair felt/reacted to the products, tools and methods used.

1. _____
2. _____
3. _____
4. _____
5. _____
6. _____
7. _____
8. _____
9. _____
10. _____
11. _____
12. _____
13. _____
14. _____
15. _____

What was the intention for your hair?

_____
_____

How did it turn out based on this expectation?

_____
_____

Learning points for next time:

My Hair:
Looks: /10
Feels: /10

Wash Day

Date: _____

Reason for washing: Routine | Dry | Product Build Up

Other: _____

Home | Salon/Stylist: _____

Wet Process

	Product(s) / Tool(s) Used	Method(s) Used
Shampoo		
Conditioner		
Treatments		
Other		

Dry Process

Detangling		
Drying		
Styling		
Other		

Comments

_____

_____

_____

_____

Wash Day – The Process

The key is in the detail: Explain which products were used and their order. Include how your hair felt/reacted to the products, tools and methods used.

1. _____
2. _____
3. _____
4. _____
5. _____
6. _____
7. _____
8. _____
9. _____
10. _____
11. _____
12. _____
13. _____
14. _____
15. _____

What was the intention for your hair?

_____

_____

How did it turn out based on this expectation?

_____

_____

Learning points for next time:

My Hair:
Looks: /10
Feels: /10

Wash Day

Date: _____

Reason for washing: Routine | Dry | Product Build Up

Other: _____

Home | Salon/Stylist: _____

Wet Process

	Product(s) / Tool(s) Used	Method(s) Used
Shampoo		
Conditioner		
Treatments		
Other		

Dry Process

Detangling		
Drying		
Styling		
Other		

Comments

_____

_____

_____

_____

Wash Day – The Process

The key is in the detail: Explain which products were used and their order. Include how your hair felt/reacted to the products, tools and methods used.

1. _____
2. _____
3. _____
4. _____
5. _____
6. _____
7. _____
8. _____
9. _____
10. _____
11. _____
12. _____
13. _____
14. _____
15. _____

What was the intention for your hair?

_____

_____

How did it turn out based on this expectation?

_____

_____

Learning points for next time:

My Hair:
Looks: /10
Feels: /10

Wash Day

Date: _____

Reason for washing: Routine | Dry | Product Build Up

Other: _____

Home | Salon/Stylist: _____

Wet Process

	Product(s) / Tool(s) Used	Method(s) Used
Shampoo		
Conditioner		
Treatments		
Other		

Dry Process

Detangling		
Drying		
Styling		
Other		

Comments

_____

_____

_____

_____

Wash Day – The Process

The key is in the detail: Explain which products were used and their order. Include how your hair felt/reacted to the products, tools and methods used.

1. _____
2. _____
3. _____
4. _____
5. _____
6. _____
7. _____
8. _____
9. _____
10. _____
11. _____
12. _____
13. _____
14. _____
15. _____

What was the intention for your hair?

_____
_____

How did it turn out based on this expectation?

_____
_____

Learning points for next time:

My Hair:
Looks: /10
Feels: /10

Wash Day

Date: _____

Reason for washing: Routine | Dry | Product Build Up

Other: _____

Home | Salon/Stylist: _____

Wet Process

	Product(s) / Tool(s) Used	Method(s) Used
Shampoo		
Conditioner		
Treatments		
Other		

Dry Process

Detangling		
Drying		
Styling		
Other		

Comments

_____

_____

_____

_____

Wash Day – The Process

The key is in the detail: Explain which products were used and their order. Include how your hair felt/reacted to the products, tools and methods used.

1. _____
2. _____
3. _____
4. _____
5. _____
6. _____
7. _____
8. _____
9. _____
10. _____
11. _____
12. _____
13. _____
14. _____
15. _____

What was the intention for your hair?

_____

_____

How did it turn out based on this expectation?

_____

_____

Learning points for next time:

My Hair:
Looks: /10
Feels: /10

Wash Day

Date: _____

Reason for washing: Routine | Dry | Product Build Up

Other: _____

Home | Salon/Stylist: _____

Wet Process

	Product(s) / Tool(s) Used	Method(s) Used
Shampoo		
Conditioner		
Treatments		
Other		

Dry Process

Detangling		
Drying		
Styling		
Other		

Comments

_____

_____

_____

_____

Wash Day – The Process

The key is in the detail: Explain which products were used and their order. Include how your hair felt/reacted to the products, tools and methods used.

1. _____
2. _____
3. _____
4. _____
5. _____
6. _____
7. _____
8. _____
9. _____
10. _____
11. _____
12. _____
13. _____
14. _____
15. _____

What was the intention for your hair?

_____

_____

How did it turn out based on this expectation?

_____

_____

Learning points for next time:

My Hair:
Looks: /10
Feels: /10

Wash Day   Date: _____

Reason for washing: Routine | Dry | Product Build Up

Other: _____

Home | Salon/Stylist: _____

Wet Process

	Product(s) / Tool(s) Used	Method(s) Used
Shampoo		
Conditioner		
Treatments		
Other		

Dry Process

Detangling		
Drying		
Styling		
Other		

Comments

_____

_____

_____

_____

Wash Day – The Process

The key is in the detail: Explain which products were used and their order. Include how your hair felt/reacted to the products, tools and methods used.

1. _____
2. _____
3. _____
4. _____
5. _____
6. _____
7. _____
8. _____
9. _____
10. _____
11. _____
12. _____
13. _____
14. _____
15. _____

What was the intention for your hair?

_____

_____

How did it turn out based on this expectation?

_____

_____

Learning points for next time:

My Hair:
Looks: /10
Feels: /10

Wash Day

Date: _____

Reason for washing: Routine | Dry | Product Build Up

Other: _____

Home | Salon/Stylist: _____

Wet Process

	Product(s) / Tool(s) Used	Method(s) Used
Shampoo		
Conditioner		
Treatments		
Other		

Dry Process

Detangling		
Drying		
Styling		
Other		

Comments

_____

_____

_____

_____

Wash Day – The Process

The key is in the detail: Explain which products were used and their order. Include how your hair felt/reacted to the products, tools and methods used.

1. _____
2. _____
3. _____
4. _____
5. _____
6. _____
7. _____
8. _____
9. _____
10. _____
11. _____
12. _____
13. _____
14. _____
15. _____

What was the intention for your hair?

_____

_____

How did it turn out based on this expectation?

_____

_____

Learning points for next time:

My Hair:
Looks: /10
Feels: /10

Wash Day

Date: _____

Reason for washing: Routine | Dry | Product Build Up

Other: _____

Home | Salon/Stylist: _____

Wet Process

	Product(s) / Tool(s) Used	Method(s) Used
Shampoo		
Conditioner		
Treatments		
Other		

Dry Process

Detangling		
Drying		
Styling		
Other		

Comments

_____

_____

_____

_____

Wash Day – The Process

The key is in the detail: Explain which products were used and their order. Include how your hair felt/reacted to the products, tools and methods used.

1. _____
2. _____
3. _____
4. _____
5. _____
6. _____
7. _____
8. _____
9. _____
10. _____
11. _____
12. _____
13. _____
14. _____
15. _____

What was the intention for your hair?

_____

_____

How did it turn out based on this expectation?

_____

_____

Learning points for next time:

My Hair:
Looks: /10
Feels: /10

Wash Day

Date: _____

Reason for washing: Routine | Dry | Product Build Up

Other: _____

Home | Salon/Stylist: _____

Wet Process

	Product(s) / Tool(s) Used	Method(s) Used
Shampoo		
Conditioner		
Treatments		
Other		

Dry Process

Detangling		
Drying		
Styling		
Other		

Comments

_____

_____

_____

_____

Wash Day – The Process

The key is in the detail: Explain which products were used and their order. Include how your hair felt/reacted to the products, tools and methods used.

1. _____
2. _____
3. _____
4. _____
5. _____
6. _____
7. _____
8. _____
9. _____
10. _____
11. _____
12. _____
13. _____
14. _____
15. _____

What was the intention for your hair?

_____
_____

How did it turn out based on this expectation?

_____
_____

Learning points for next time:

My Hair:
Looks: /10
Feels: /10

Wash Day

Date: _____

Reason for washing: Routine | Dry | Product Build Up

Other: _____

Home | Salon/Stylist: _____

Wet Process

	Product(s) / Tool(s) Used	Method(s) Used
Shampoo		
Conditioner		
Treatments		
Other		

Dry Process

Detangling		
Drying		
Styling		
Other		

Comments

_____

_____

_____

_____

Wash Day – The Process

The key is in the detail: Explain which products were used and their order. Include how your hair felt/reacted to the products, tools and methods used.

1. _____
2. _____
3. _____
4. _____
5. _____
6. _____
7. _____
8. _____
9. _____
10. _____
11. _____
12. _____
13. _____
14. _____
15. _____

What was the intention for your hair?

_____

_____

How did it turn out based on this expectation?

_____

_____

Learning points for next time:

My Hair:
Looks: /10
Feels: /10

wash day

Date: _____

Reason for washing: Routine | Dry | Product Build Up

Other: _____

Home | Salon/Stylist: _____

Wet Process

	Product(s) / Tool(s) Used	Method(s) Used
Shampoo		
Conditioner		
Treatments		
Other		

Dry Process

Detangling		
Drying		
Styling		
Other		

Comments

_____

_____

_____

_____

Wash Day – The Process

The key is in the detail: Explain which products were used and their order. Include how your hair felt/reacted to the products, tools and methods used.

1. _____
2. _____
3. _____
4. _____
5. _____
6. _____
7. _____
8. _____
9. _____
10. _____
11. _____
12. _____
13. _____
14. _____
15. _____

What was the intention for your hair?

_____

_____

How did it turn out based on this expectation?

_____

_____

Learning points for next time:

My Hair:
Looks: /10
Feels: /10

Chemical Processing   Date: _____

Home | Salon/Stylist: _____

Type of Process: _____

Reason for Application: _____

Product Used: _____

Applied to: Full Head | Roots | Other: _____

Application Time: _____   Processing Time: _____

Total Time: _____

Applied to _____ first e.g. back left quarter

Applied to _____ last

Pre-Process

	Product(s) / Tool(s) Used	Method(s) Used
Hair Preparation		
Other		
Other		

Application method and comments

_____

_____

_____

_____

_____

_____

_____

Chemical Processing Continued...

Wet Process

Shampoo		
Conditioner		
Treatments		
Other		

Dry Process

Detangling		
Drying		
Styling		
Other		

How did your hair turn out?

_____

_____

_____

_____

_____

Learning points for next time:

Chemical Processing   Date: _____

Home | Salon/Stylist: _____

Type of Process: _____

Reason for Application: _____

Product Used: _____

Applied to: Full Head | Roots | Other: _____

Application Time: _____   Processing Time: _____

Total Time: _____

Applied to _____ first e.g. back left quarter

Applied to _____ last

Pre-Process

	Product(s) / Tool(s) Used	Method(s) Used
Hair Preparation		
Other		
Other		

Application method and comments

_____

_____

_____

_____

_____

_____

_____

Chemical Processing Continued...

Wet Process

Shampoo		
Conditioner		
Treatments		
Other		

Dry Process

Detangling		
Drying		
Styling		
Other		

How did your hair turn out?

_____

_____

_____

_____

_____

Learning points for next time:

Chemical Processing   Date: _____

Home | Salon/Stylist: _____

Type of Process: _____

Reason for Application: _____

Product Used: _____

Applied to: Full Head | Roots | Other: _____

Application Time: _____   Processing Time: _____

Total Time: _____

Applied to _____ first e.g. back left quarter

Applied to _____ last

Pre-Process

	Product(s) / Tool(s) Used	Method(s) Used
Hair Preparation		
Other		
Other		

Application method and comments

_____

_____

_____

_____

_____

_____

_____

Chemical Processing Continued...

Wet Process

Shampoo		
Conditioner		
Treatments		
Other		

Dry Process

Detangling		
Drying		
Styling		
Other		

How did your hair turn out?

_____

_____

_____

_____

_____

Learning points for next time:

Chemical Processing   Date: _____

Home | Salon/Stylist: _____

Type of Process: _____

Reason for Application: _____

Product Used: _____

Applied to: Full Head | Roots | Other: _____

Application Time: _____   Processing Time: _____

Total Time: _____

Applied to _____ first e.g. back left quarter

Applied to _____ last

Pre-Process

	Product(s) / Tool(s) Used	Method(s) Used
Hair Preparation		
Other		
Other		

Application method and comments

_____

_____

_____

_____

_____

_____

_____

Chemical Processing Continued...

Wet Process

Shampoo		
Conditioner		
Treatments		
Other		

Dry Process

Detangling		
Drying		
Styling		
Other		

How did your hair turn out?

_____

_____

_____

_____

_____

Learning points for next time:

Chemical Processing   Date: _____

Home | Salon/Stylist: _____

Type of Process: _____

Reason for Application: _____

Product Used: _____

Applied to: Full Head | Roots | Other: _____

Application Time: _____   Processing Time: _____

Total Time: _____

Applied to _____ first e.g. back left quarter

Applied to _____ last

Pre-Process

	Product(s) / Tool(s) Used	Method(s) Used
Hair Preparation		
Other		
Other		

Application method and comments

_____

_____

_____

_____

_____

_____

_____

Chemical Processing Continued...

Wet Process

Shampoo		
Conditioner		
Treatments		
Other		

Dry Process

Detangling		
Drying		
Styling		
Other		

How did your hair turn out?

_____

_____

_____

_____

_____

Learning points for next time:

Chemical Processing   Date: _____

Home | Salon/Stylist: _____

Type of Process: _____

Reason for Application: _____

Product Used: _____

Applied to: Full Head | Roots | Other: _____

Application Time: _____   Processing Time: _____

Total Time: _____

Applied to _____ first e.g. back left quarter

Applied to _____ last

Pre-Process

	Product(s) / Tool(s) Used	Method(s) Used
Hair Preparation		
Other		
Other		

Application method and comments

_____
_____
_____
_____
_____
_____
_____

Chemical Processing Continued...

Wet Process

Shampoo		
Conditioner		
Treatments		
Other		

Dry Process

Detangling		
Drying		
Styling		
Other		

How did your hair turn out?

_____

_____

_____

_____

_____

Learning points for next time:

Chemical Processing   Date: _____

Home | Salon/Stylist: _____

Type of Process: _____

Reason for Application: _____

Product Used: _____

Applied to: Full Head | Roots | Other: _____

Application Time: _____   Processing Time: _____

Total Time: _____

Applied to _____ first e.g. back left quarter

Applied to _____ last

Pre-Process

	Product(s) / Tool(s) Used	Method(s) Used
Hair Preparation		
Other		
Other		

Application method and comments

_____
_____
_____
_____
_____
_____
_____

Chemical Processing Continued...

Wet Process

Shampoo		
Conditioner		
Treatments		
Other		

Dry Process

Detangling		
Drying		
Styling		
Other		

How did your hair turn out?

_____

_____

_____

_____

_____

Learning points for next time:

Chemical Processing   Date: _____

Home | Salon/Stylist: _____

Type of Process: _____

Reason for Application: _____

Product Used: _____

Applied to: Full Head | Roots | Other: _____

Application Time: _____   Processing Time: _____

Total Time: _____

Applied to _____ first e.g. back left quarter

Applied to _____ last

Pre-Process

	Product(s) / Tool(s) Used	Method(s) Used
Hair Preparation		
Other		
Other		

Application method and comments

_____

_____

_____

_____

_____

_____

_____

Chemical Processing Continued...

Wet Process

Shampoo		
Conditioner		
Treatments		
Other		

Dry Process

Detangling		
Drying		
Styling		
Other		

How did your hair turn out?

_____

_____

_____

_____

_____

Learning points for next time:

Protective Styles

Install Date	Hair Prep	Products/Tools	Style	Removal Date	Post Hair Condition
Notes					
Notes					
Notes					
Notes					
Notes					
Notes					

Protective Styles

Install Date	Hair Prep	Products/ Tools	Style	Removal Date	Post Hair Condition
Notes					
Notes					
Notes					
Notes					
Notes					
Notes					

Cuts and Trims

Date	Cut or Trim	Reason	Hair Prep + Wet/Dry	CM/IN Cut Off	Products/ Tools
Notes					
Notes					
Notes					
Notes					
Notes					
Notes					

Cuts and Trims

Date	Cut or Trim	Reason	Hair Prep + Wet/Dry	CM/IN Cut Off	Products/ Tools
Notes					
Notes					
Notes					
Notes					
Notes					
Notes					

Supplements

Note the supplements you are currently taking - remember to log usage on the daily hair tracker

Start Date	Supplement	Dosage	Stop Date	Results/Side Effect/Notes

3 Month Check In   Date: _____

Hair Thickness: Fine | Thin | Thick | Coarse

Hair Density: Low | Medium | High

Hair Porosity: Low | Medium | High

Hair Condition: Healthy | Damaged | Shiny | Dull | Soft

Dry | Brittle | Spongy | Rough | Smooth | Frizzy | _____

What have you changed in your routine recently and how may it have affected your hair?

_____

_____

_____

_____

Additional Comments

_____

_____

_____

Hair Length (inches):

Top: _____   Crown: _____   Nape: _____

Above Ear (Left): _____   Above Ear (Right): _____

Below Ear (Left): _____   Below Ear (Right): _____

Problem Areas	Achievements

6 Month Check In   Date: _____

Hair Thickness: Fine | Thin | Thick | Coarse

Hair Density: Low | Medium | High

Hair Porosity: Low | Medium | High

Hair Condition: Healthy | Damaged | Shiny | Dull | Soft

Dry | Brittle | Spongy | Rough | Smooth | Frizzy | _____

What have you changed in your routine recently and how may it have affected your hair?

_____

_____

_____

_____

Additional Comments

_____

_____

_____

Hair Length (inches):

Top: _____   Crown: _____   Nape: _____

Above Ear (Left): _____   Above Ear (Right): _____

Below Ear (Left): _____   Below Ear (Right): _____

Problem Areas	Achievements

9 Month Check In   Date: _____

Hair Thickness: Fine | Thin | Thick | Coarse

Hair Density: Low | Medium | High

Hair Porosity: Low | Medium | High

Hair Condition: Healthy | Damaged | Shiny | Dull | Soft

Dry | Brittle | Spongy | Rough | Smooth | Frizzy | _____

What have you changed in your routine recently and how may it have affected your hair?

_____

_____

_____

_____

Additional Comments

_____

_____

_____

Hair Length (inches):

Top: _____ Crown: _____ Nape: _____

Above Ear (Left): _____ Above Ear (Right): _____

Below Ear (Left): _____ Below Ear (Right): _____

Problem Areas	Achievements

Final Check In   Date: _____

Hair Thickness: Fine | Thin | Thick | Coarse
Hair Density: Low | Medium | High
Hair Porosity: Low | Medium | High
Hair Condition: Healthy | Damaged | Shiny | Dull | Soft
Dry | Brittle | Spongy | Rough | Smooth | Frizzy | _____

How would you describe your hair now? _____
_____
_____

Additional Comments
_____
_____

Areas needing improvement:

_____
| |
| |
| |
|_____|

Hair Length (inches):

Top: _____   Crown: _____   Nape: _____

Above Ear (Left): _____   Above Ear (Right): _____

Below Ear (Left): _____   Below Ear (Right): _____

Improved Areas:

| |
| |
| |
|_____|

final Check In continued...

This worked best:

	Daily	Twice Weekly	Weekly	Twice Monthly	Monthly	Less
Shampoo						
Condition						
Deep Condition						
Moisturize						
Blow Dry						
Flat Iron						
Trim						
Cut						
Protective Style						
Other						

Since you started, how has your routine changed?

_____

_____

What changes has benefited your hair the most?

_____

_____

How will you continue to build on your hair regime?

_____

_____

Ultimate Hair Care Regime

Flick through the 'Wash Day – The Process' pages of this journal and find out the scores in the 'My Hair' section.

Common themes for my lowest scoring wash days:

_____

_____

Common themes for my highest scoring wash days:

_____

_____

What was your most common reason for washing?

_____

What products were used on the highest scoring days:

Shampoo: _____ Conditioner: _____

Treatments: _____ Tools: _____

Which methods were used on these wash days:

Detangling: _____ Drying: _____

Styling: _____

What has changed from the 'Hair Profile' to now?

_____

_____

_____

Did you keep your hair moisturized between washes?

_____

Comments

_____

_____

Ultimate Hair Care Regime Continued...

Explain the routines and products that work well for your hair based on the new information you have.

Washing

Drying

Detangling

Styling

Moisturizing

Other

Notes

Printed in Great Britain
by Amazon